YAKALOU MEDIA

Questions to Ask Before Having a Baby

100 Questions To Ask Yourself Before Having a Baby

First edition

This book was professionally typeset on Reedsy.
Find out more at reedsy.com

Contents

Disclaimer   v

I   Setting The Stage

1   Introduction   3
2   The 5 Rules to Get the Most Out of This Book   5
3   Word of Warning Before We Start   8
4   How to Use This Book Your Way   10

II   Your 100 Questions To Ask Before Having
A Baby

5   Chapter 1: Health and Wellness   15
6   Exercise #1   19
7   Chapter 2: The Financial Part of It   20
8   Exercise #2   24
9   Chapter 3: Relationship and Support   25
10 Exercise #3   29
11 Chapter 4: Parenting Styles   30
12 Exercise #4   34
13 Chapter 5: Work and Career   35
14 Exercise #5   39
15 Chapter 6: Living Arrangements   40
16 Exercise #6   44

17	Chapter 7: Emotional Preparedness	45
18	Exercise #7	49
19	Chapter 8: Childcare and Education	50
20	Exercise #8	54
21	Chapter 9: Lifestyle Changes	55
22	Exercise #9	59
23	Chapter 10: Emergency and Contingency Planning	60
24	Exercise #10	64
25	Now WHAT? You May Ask	65
26	Conclusion	68

Disclaimer

This book is designed to provide information only. This information is provided and sold with the knowledge that the publisher and author do not offer any legal or other professional advice. In the case of a need for any such expertise, consult with the appropriate professional.

This book does not contain all the information available on the subject. This book has not been created to be specific to any individual's or organization's situation or needs. Every effort has been made to make this book as accurate as possible. However, there may be typographical and/or content errors. Therefore, this book should serve only as a general guide, not as the ultimate source of subject information.

This book contains information that might be dated and is intended only to educate and entertain. Regarding any loss or damage allegedly suffered or alleged to have occurred as a result of the information in this book, either directly or indirectly, the author and publisher shall have no liability or responsibility to any person or entity.

I

Setting The Stage

1

Introduction

Bringing a new life into the world is one of the most profound decisions you will ever make. But are you truly ready? Parenthood is not just about the joy of holding a tiny, fragile baby in your arms. It's about a lifetime of responsibility, love, sacrifice, and endless questions. Before you take this life-changing step, have you asked yourself the right questions?

What does it mean to be ready for a baby? Is it just about financial stability, or does it go deeper into your emotional and physical well-being? Have you and your partner talked about how a child will change your relationship, your daily routines, and even your future dreams? These questions might seem overwhelming, but they are essential to ensuring that you are prepared for the journey ahead.

Many couples dive into parenthood without fully understanding the challenges and joys that come with it. They might focus on the excitement of a new baby without considering the sleepless nights, the financial strain, or the impact on their careers and social lives. Have you thought about how your life will change when you bring a child into it? Are you ready to make the sacrifices needed, or are you prepared to face the unexpected?

Before you embark on this incredible journey, it's important to pause and reflect. Asking yourself the right questions now can save you from potential regrets later. Are you and your partner on the same page about parenting styles, work-life balance, and the kind of future you want for your child? These are conversations that need to happen before a baby arrives, not after.

This book is here to guide you through the essential questions you should consider before having a baby. It's not about scaring you or making you doubt your decision. Instead, it's about helping you prepare—mentally, emotionally, and practically—for one of the biggest adventures of your life. Are you ready to explore these questions together?

In the pages that follow, you'll find questions that cover everything from your health and financial readiness to your relationship dynamics and lifestyle changes. Each question is designed to make you think deeply about your readiness for parenthood. So, take your time with each one. Discuss them with your partner. Reflect on your answers. Are you prepared to make informed decisions that will shape your future and the future of your child?

Let's begin this journey together. Are you ready to ask yourself the most important questions before bringing a new life into the world?

2

The 5 Rules to Get the Most Out of This Book

Before you dive into the questions and reflections in this book, it's important to understand how to get the most out of what's inside. You're about to embark on a journey that could shape the rest of your life. But how do you ensure that this journey is as meaningful and useful as possible? Let's start by laying down five simple rules that will help you make the most of every page.

Rule 1: Be Honest with Yourself

The first and most important rule is honesty. Are you truly being open with yourself as you answer these questions? This book is meant to help you reflect deeply on your readiness for parenthood, but that only works if you're willing to face your true feelings and thoughts. Sometimes, the truth might be uncomfortable or challenging. Are you ready to confront that? Remember, the more honest you are with yourself, the more clarity you'll gain.

Rule 2: Take Your Time

This isn't a race. There's no prize for finishing quickly. Have you ever rushed through something important only to realize later that you missed crucial details? To get the most out of this book, give yourself the time to think, reflect, and discuss each question. Parenting is a lifetime commitment; shouldn't the decision to start that journey be given careful thought? So, slow down, take breaks when needed, and allow yourself the space to process your thoughts fully.

Rule 3: Communicate with Your Partner

Parenting is a team effort, and this book is designed to be a conversation starter. Have you shared your thoughts and concerns with your partner as you go through the questions? Open, honest communication with your partner is key to aligning your goals, expectations, and dreams for the future. After all, you're in this together. Use this book as a tool to strengthen your bond and ensure you're both on the same page.

Rule 4: Keep an Open Mind

It's easy to think we know all the answers, but do we really? This book might bring up ideas or concerns you haven't considered before. Are you willing to explore new perspectives? Keeping an open mind means being ready to reassess your beliefs and being flexible enough to adapt to new information. Parenthood is full of surprises, and being open to learning and growing will only make you better prepared.

Rule 5: Revisit and Reflect

The final rule is to revisit and reflect on your answers. Life is constantly changing, and so are you. Have your thoughts or feelings shifted since you first answered a question? It's important to go back, look at your previous answers, and see if they still hold true. This book isn't just a one-time read; it's a resource you can return to as your journey toward parenthood evolves. Reflection helps you stay grounded and aware of your growth.

By following these five rules, you'll maximize the value of this book. It's not just about answering questions; it's about engaging deeply with your own thoughts and emotions, communicating effectively with your partner, and staying open to what you learn along the way. Are you ready to embark on this journey with an open heart and mind? If so, these rules will guide you toward making the most informed and thoughtful decisions for your future.

<h1 style="text-align:center">3</h1>

Word of Warning Before We Start

Before we dive into the questions and reflections in this book, let's pause for a moment. Are you ready to face the reality of what lies ahead? This isn't just a guide filled with questions; it's a mirror that will reflect your true feelings, your fears, your hopes, and maybe even your doubts. Before you turn the page, there's something important you need to understand.

The journey you're about to begin is not always going to be easy. Have you ever faced a tough decision, only to find that the more you thought about it, the more complex it became? That's exactly what you might experience as you go through this book. The questions we'll explore together are designed to challenge you. They might bring up emotions you didn't expect or force you to reconsider things you thought you were sure about. Are you prepared for that?

It's important to remember that there are no right or wrong answers here. Every question is an opportunity to dig deeper, to explore your inner thoughts and feelings. But with that exploration comes a warning: you may uncover truths that are difficult to face. Are you willing to confront those truths? You might realize that you're not as ready as you thought, or that there are areas of your life that need more attention before you take the leap into parenthood. It's okay to feel uncertain or even scared. That's part of the process.

This book isn't just about preparation; it's about introspection. But introspection can be uncomfortable. Have you ever looked at yourself in the mirror and really seen what's there, beyond the surface? That's what this book will ask you to do. It will ask you to examine your relationships, your finances, your mental and physical health, and even your dreams for the future. Some of these reflections might be tough to swallow. But would you rather face these challenges now or be blindsided by them later?

As you embark on this journey, remember that it's okay to feel vulnerable. It's okay to have doubts. In fact, those doubts are a sign that you're taking this seriously. Are you ready to embrace the discomfort, knowing that it will lead to greater clarity and understanding? This process is about building a solid foundation for the future, and sometimes that means tearing down old walls before you can start anew.

So, consider this your word of warning: this book will challenge you. It will make you think, feel, and reflect in ways you might not expect. But isn't that exactly what you want before making one of the biggest decisions of your life? If you're ready to face the hard questions and the honest answers, then you're ready to begin. This journey won't always be easy, but it will be worth it. Are you ready to take the first step?

4

How to Use This Book Your Way

You might be wondering, do I need to read every single page of this book? The simple answer is: no, you don't. This book is designed to be as flexible as you need it to be. Life is busy, and sometimes you don't have the time—or the patience—to read a book cover to cover. And that's okay. You can pick it up whenever you have a moment, and dive into the sections that speak to you the most at that time.

Each question in this book stands on its own, offering insight into a different aspect of preparing for parenthood. Maybe today you're thinking about your finances, and you want to focus on those questions. Or perhaps a conversation with your partner has brought up concerns about your relationship, and you want to explore that more deeply. You can easily skip to the relevant sections without feeling like you've missed something essential. Isn't it nice to have that freedom?

Think of this book as a toolbox, where each question is a tool that you can use when you need it. Just like you wouldn't use every tool in a toolbox for every project, you don't need to engage with every question in this book all at once. Are you more comfortable taking things one step at a time? Then flip through the pages, see what catches your eye, and start there. You're in control.

Remember, this book is here to help you, not overwhelm you. Whether you're skimming through or diving deep into every detail, you're doing it right. There's no wrong way to use this book. So go ahead—trust your instincts, skip around, and find the questions that resonate with you today. Tomorrow, you might find yourself drawn to different sections. And that's perfectly fine.

II

Your 100 Questions To Ask Before Having A Baby

5

Chapter 1: Health and Wellness

Sarah had always dreamed of becoming a mother. In her early thirties, with a stable career and a loving partner, she felt the time was finally right. But as she began thinking seriously about starting a family, doubts crept in. Sarah wasn't sure if her body was truly ready for the demands of pregnancy. She had never given much thought to her health beyond the occasional cold or minor aches. Now, the stakes were higher, and she knew she needed to get serious about her well-being.

One morning, Sarah sat in her kitchen, sipping tea, and scrolling through an article about prenatal health. The more she read, the more she realized how much she didn't know. What if there was something in her medical history that could complicate pregnancy? Should she be eating differently? What about her mental health? These were questions she had never considered before.

As Sarah pondered these thoughts, she decided to take the first step by scheduling a check-up with her doctor. The appointment was eye-opening. Her doctor talked her through the importance of a full medical evaluation before trying to conceive. Sarah learned that even minor issues, like a vitamin deficiency or unmanaged stress, could have significant effects on her ability to get pregnant and on her pregnancy itself.

This visit sparked more questions in Sarah's mind. Was she getting enough of the right nutrients? How would her body handle the changes that come with pregnancy? And importantly, was she mentally prepared for this life-changing journey? She realized that while pregnancy is a natural process, it demands more from the body and mind than she had ever considered.

Preparing for pregnancy is much more than just deciding to have a baby. It's about understanding your body's current state, addressing any health concerns, and making sure you are in the best possible shape—both physically and mentally. Sarah began to appreciate that this preparation phase is crucial not just for her, but for the future well-being of her baby too.

Reflecting on her own habits, Sarah started making small but significant changes. She swapped out her afternoon coffee for a nutritious smoothie, took up yoga to manage stress, and made sure she was getting enough sleep. These adjustments, though simple, helped her feel more in control and confident in her journey toward motherhood.

As you read this, you might find yourself in a similar place as Sarah. You're ready to start a family, but you're unsure if your body is truly prepared for the task. It's normal to have these questions, and it's important to take the time to answer them before embarking on the journey of pregnancy. Your health and wellness are the foundation for a healthy pregnancy and baby.

So, where do you start? Begin by asking yourself some fundamental questions about your health. Are you aware of any medical conditions that could affect pregnancy? Have you discussed your plans with a healthcare provider? What lifestyle changes can you make to better prepare your body? And just as crucially, how will you ensure that your mental health is taken care of during this process?

These questions are not just about ticking off a checklist. They are about understanding and caring for yourself in a way that prepares you for one of life's most significant changes. By taking the time to explore these aspects of your health, you are setting the stage for a smoother, healthier pregnancy.

To help guide you, here are 10 key questions to consider as you prepare for this important phase of your life. After reflecting on these, try the practical exercise to deepen your understanding of your current health and what you might need to work on.

Key Questions:

1. Have I had a full medical check-up recently?
2. What lifestyle changes should I make to prepare my body for pregnancy?
3. Are there any pre-existing medical conditions that could affect pregnancy?
4. Am I getting enough nutrients, like folic acid, in my diet?
5. Should I take any prenatal vitamins or supplements?
6. Do I have a plan to manage stress and mental health during pregnancy?
7. How does my family's medical history impact my pregnancy?
8. What are the risks associated with my age and pregnancy?
9. Have I discussed my pregnancy plans with my doctor or healthcare provider?
10. Do I understand the stages of pregnancy and the changes

my body will go through?

6

Exercise #1

Practical Exercise:

Create a Personal Wellness Plan: Take a moment to write down your current health habits, including your diet, exercise routine, sleep patterns, and stress management strategies. Next, identify any areas that could use improvement, such as eating more vegetables, exercising more regularly, or finding new ways to relax. Set small, realistic goals for each area and plan how you will achieve them. For example, you might decide to add an extra serving of vegetables to your meals each day or start a 10-minute daily meditation practice. This plan will be your roadmap to better health as you prepare for pregnancy.

Chapter 2: The Financial Part of It

When Rachel and Tom first decided to start a family, they were over the moon with excitement. They imagined the joys of parenthood—the first smiles, tiny clothes, and all the sweet moments in between. But as they sat down one evening to look at their finances, reality started to set in. How would they afford everything a baby needs? What would happen to their savings? And how could they prepare for the unexpected costs that might arise?

Rachel had always been careful with money, but the idea of budgeting for a baby felt overwhelming. Diapers, clothes, a crib, daycare—the list of expenses seemed endless. She realized that their usual monthly budget would need a serious overhaul. As they began to talk it over, Tom confessed that he hadn't thought much about the financial side of things. He figured they'd just make it work, somehow. But Rachel wasn't so sure. She knew that having a solid financial plan was crucial, not just for peace of mind, but to ensure they could provide the best for their future child.

This conversation led them to seek advice from friends who

were already parents. What they learned was eye-opening. The cost of raising a child starts long before the baby arrives and continues to grow as they get older. Rachel and Tom began to see that preparing for a baby wasn't just about buying cute outfits and toys—it was about creating a financial cushion that would allow them to handle whatever came their way.

Rachel began to dig deeper into their finances. She started by listing all the potential expenses: prenatal care, hospital bills, baby gear, and ongoing costs like food, clothing, and childcare. She quickly realized that they needed to start saving immediately, and more aggressively than they had been. But saving was just one piece of the puzzle. Rachel knew they needed a budget that accounted for both their current expenses and the additional costs a baby would bring.

As they started to rework their budget, Rachel and Tom faced some tough decisions. They realized that they might need to cut back on dining out, postpone that vacation they'd been dreaming about, and rethink their shopping habits. It wasn't easy, but they both agreed that the sacrifices were worth it if it meant they could give their child a secure start in life.

In addition to saving and budgeting, Rachel began to explore other financial questions. Should they invest in a college fund? Did they have enough life insurance to cover potential emergencies? And how would Tom's paternity leave affect their income? These questions led to more discussions, each one bringing them closer to a clear financial plan.

For Rachel and Tom, the process of financially preparing for a baby was both challenging and enlightening. It required them to take a hard look at their spending, make necessary adjustments, and plan for the future with care and intention. They learned that financial readiness is not just about having enough money in the bank; it's about understanding where your money goes, making informed decisions, and being prepared for the unexpected.

As you read this, you might be wondering how to start preparing financially for a baby. You're not alone in feeling overwhelmed by the costs, but with some careful planning, you can build a solid financial foundation for your growing family. Start by asking yourself key questions: How much do you need to save? What are your current spending habits, and where can you make cuts? How will your income change once the baby arrives?

By answering these questions, you can begin to create a financial plan that works for you. Remember, the goal is not to have everything figured out perfectly but to ensure that you are financially prepared for this new chapter in your life. It's about making sure that when the time comes, you can focus on enjoying parenthood without constantly worrying about money.

To help you get started, here are 10 essential questions to consider as you prepare for the financial aspects of having a baby. After you reflect on these, try the practical exercise to help you create a budget that takes into account both your current needs and the future needs of your child.

Key Questions:

1. How much money do I need to save before having a baby?
2. Have I researched the costs of prenatal care and delivery?
3. What is the cost of baby essentials like diapers, clothing, and a crib?
4. How will having a baby impact our household budget?

5. Should we consider life insurance or an emergency fund for our family?
6. How much will childcare cost, and how will we afford it?
7. What are the long-term financial responsibilities of raising a child?
8. Should we start a college savings plan for the baby?
9. How will maternity/paternity leave affect our income?
10. Have we reviewed our health insurance to cover pregnancy and childbirth?

8

Exercise #2

Practical Exercise:

Create a Baby Budget: Start by listing all your current monthly expenses, including rent or mortgage, utilities, groceries, and entertainment. Next, add in the estimated costs associated with having a baby, such as diapers, formula, baby gear, and daycare. Don't forget to include one-time expenses like a crib or car seat. Compare this new budget to your current income and savings. Identify areas where you can cut back or save more, and set a realistic savings goal for each month leading up to the baby's arrival. This exercise will help you see exactly where your money is going and how to plan for the future.

Chapter 3: Relationship and Support

Emily and Jake had been together for seven years when they decided to have a baby. Their relationship had always been strong; they communicated well, supported each other's goals, and shared a deep love. But as they started planning for a baby, Emily began to worry about how this new chapter might change their relationship. Would they still find time for each other? How would they navigate the inevitable stress and exhaustion that comes with parenting? These thoughts kept Emily awake at night, even as she eagerly anticipated becoming a mother.

One evening, over a quiet dinner, Emily brought up her concerns. She was nervous, afraid that discussing these fears might make them real, but she knew it was important to talk about them. Jake listened carefully, nodding in agreement. He admitted that he had similar worries. Their relationship had always been their anchor, and the thought of it being strained by the challenges of parenthood was unsettling.

This honest conversation was a turning point for them. They realized that preparing for a baby wasn't just about buying the right gear or setting up a nursery—it was about strengthening their relationship and ensuring they were ready to face the ups and downs of parenthood together. They started to explore what their roles would be as parents, how they would share responsibilities, and most importantly, how they would continue to nurture their relationship.

Emily and Jake decided to create a plan to stay connected as a couple, even in the midst of sleepless nights and diaper changes. They made a pact to have a weekly date night, no matter how tired they were. They also agreed to keep communication open, to talk about their feelings and concerns without judgment. These small commitments made them feel more united and prepared for the changes ahead.

But they knew that it wasn't just about their relationship. They would also need support from their family and friends. Emily had always been close to her mother, and she knew she would rely on her for advice and help when the baby arrived. Jake, on the other hand, wasn't as comfortable asking for help, but he understood that having a strong support system was crucial.

They began to reach out to their loved ones, letting them know about their plans and asking if they would be there to support them. The responses were overwhelmingly positive. Their friends and family were excited to help in any way they could, offering to babysit, bring meals, or just be there to listen. This support network gave Emily and Jake a sense of security, knowing they wouldn't have to navigate parenthood alone.

As they continued to prepare, Emily and Jake realized that their relationship and support system would be the foundation of their parenting journey. They understood that while the challenges would be real, having each other and the support of those around them would make all the difference.

If you're planning to have a baby, it's essential to consider how this major life change will affect your relationship and the support you'll need. It's not just about the love you have for each other; it's about how you communicate, share responsibilities, and lean on your support network. How will you ensure that your relationship remains strong? Who can you turn to for help, and how will you ask for it?

As you think about these questions, remember that preparing for a baby is not just a physical and financial journey but an emotional and relational one as well. Strengthening your relationship and building a solid support system can help you face the challenges of parenthood with confidence and resilience.

To help guide your thoughts, here are 10 key questions to consider about your relationship and support network. After reflecting on these, try the practical exercise to further strengthen your connection with your partner and identify your support resources.

Key Questions:

1. How do we feel about becoming parents at this stage of our relationship?
2. What are our expectations for each other as co-parents?
3. How will we handle disagreements about parenting decisions?
4. Do we have a support system of family and friends to help us?
5. How will our relationship change after the baby is born?
6. What roles will each of us take on in parenting?
7. How will we manage time for ourselves and our relation-

ship?

8. Have we discussed how to share household responsibilities after the baby arrives?

9. What are our expectations about intimacy and connection post-baby?

10. How will we support each other emotionally during the challenges of parenting?

10

Exercise #3

Practical Exercise:

Strengthen Your Connection: Set aside time for a deep, un-interrupted conversation with your partner. Start by sharing your hopes and fears about becoming parents. Then, discuss how you will support each other during this transition. Talk about the specific ways you can stay connected as a couple, such as regular date nights, open communication, and sharing responsibilities. After the conversation, make a list of your top three commitments to each other. Write them down and place them somewhere visible as a reminder of your promises. This exercise will help you align your expectations and strengthen your bond as you prepare for the journey ahead.

Chapter 4: Parenting Styles

When Ava and Lucas first found out they were expecting, they were overjoyed. They spent hours daydreaming about their future child, imagining what they would look like, what their first words might be, and how they would fit into their little family. But as the weeks went by, they realized that they had never really talked about how they would parent. How would they discipline their child? What values were most important to them? And how would they handle the inevitable challenges that come with raising a child?

One evening, as they were relaxing on the couch, Ava brought up the topic. "How do you think we should raise our baby?" she asked. Lucas paused, a bit surprised by the question. He hadn't really thought about it in detail. "I guess... the way we were raised?" he replied, uncertainly. But Ava wasn't satisfied with that answer. She knew that they needed to be more intentional about their parenting approach.

This conversation opened the door to a deeper discussion about their own childhoods, their beliefs, and the kind of parents they wanted to be. Ava had grown up in a home where discipline was strict, but she also felt deeply loved and supported. Lucas, on the other hand, had a more relaxed upbringing, where he was encouraged to explore and make his own decisions from a young age. They realized that their experiences shaped their views on parenting, but they also knew they needed to find a middle ground that worked for both of them.

As they talked, Ava and Lucas started to think about the values they wanted to instill in their child. Kindness, honesty, and resilience were at the top of their list. They also discussed education—how they wanted their child to love learning, but without feeling pressured to be perfect. They both agreed that fostering a sense of curiosity and creativity was crucial, but they had different ideas on how to achieve that.

The topic of discipline was more challenging. Ava believed in setting clear boundaries and using consequences to teach lessons, while Lucas preferred a more gentle approach, focusing on communication and understanding. They realized that they would need to find a balance, blending both their styles to create a consistent and loving environment for their child.

As they continued to explore their parenting styles, they began to see the importance of being on the same page. They knew that consistency was key to raising a child who feels secure and loved. They also recognized that parenting is an evolving process, one that would require them to adapt and grow as their child developed.

Ava and Lucas decided to keep the conversation going, regularly checking in with each other about their parenting decisions. They knew that challenges would arise, but they felt confident that by discussing their values and approaches upfront, they could navigate those challenges together.

For anyone about to embark on the journey of parenthood, it's essential to think about your parenting style. How do you want to raise your child? What values are most important to you? How will you handle discipline, education, and the everyday decisions that shape your child's life? These questions are not just about the kind of parent you want to be—they're about the kind of person you want your child to become.

As you consider your parenting style, remember that there is no one-size-fits-all approach. The most important thing is to be thoughtful and intentional, to communicate openly with your partner, and to be willing to adapt as you learn and grow along with your child.

To help guide you, here are 10 key questions to consider about your parenting style. After reflecting on these, try the practical exercise to align your parenting goals with your partner and ensure you're both working toward the same vision for your family.

Key Questions:

1. What are the most important values we want to instill in our child?
2. How do we feel about different parenting styles (e.g., strict, lenient)?
3. How will we approach discipline and setting boundaries?
4. What role does religion or spirituality play in our parenting?
5. How do we feel about screen time and technology for our child?
6. How important is education, and what kind of schooling do we prefer?

7. How do we plan to teach our child about diversity and inclusion?
8. What are our thoughts on vaccinations and medical care for our child?
9. How will we handle differences in our parenting approaches?
10. How do we feel about raising a child with the influence of extended family?

12

Exercise #4

Practical Exercise:

Define Your Parenting Values: Take some time with your partner to write down the top five values you want to instill in your child. Discuss why these values are important to each of you and how you can incorporate them into your daily parenting practices. For example, if kindness is a core value, think about ways you can model and encourage kindness in your home. Then, talk about how you'll approach discipline, education, and other key aspects of parenting to support these values. This exercise will help you create a unified parenting philosophy that reflects both your beliefs and your hopes for your child's future.

Chapter 5: Work and Career

Jessica loved her job. As a project manager for a growing tech company, she thrived on the challenges and excitement that came with leading teams and delivering results. Her career was on an upward trajectory, and she had big plans for the future. But when she found out she was pregnant, Jessica's mind started racing with new questions. How would she balance her demanding career with the responsibilities of motherhood? Would she be able to take enough time off after the baby was born? And what would happen to her long-term career goals once she became a parent?

These questions kept Jessica up at night, even as she felt the joy of expecting her first child. She knew she needed to plan carefully to make sure she could continue to grow in her career while also being the kind of mother she wanted to be. But as she began to explore her options, she realized that finding the right balance wouldn't be easy.

One of the first things Jessica did was talk to her HR department about maternity leave. She was relieved to find out that her company offered generous leave options, but she still had concerns. Would taking several months off set her back in her career? How would her team manage without her? And would she be able to return to work with the same level of energy and focus?

Jessica also started to think about the logistics of balancing work and parenthood. She knew that her job often required long hours and late nights. How would she manage that with a baby at home? And what about when the baby got sick or when she needed to attend a school event? She realized that she would need a flexible plan to handle the unexpected challenges that come with being a working parent.

As Jessica considered these questions, she began to discuss her concerns with her partner, David. David was supportive and eager to share the responsibilities of parenthood, but he also had his own career to consider. They talked about how they could divide the duties of parenting, who would handle drop-offs and pick-ups, and what they would do if one of them had to travel for work. These conversations were essential in helping them create a plan that worked for both of their careers and their new family life.

Jessica also reached out to other working parents in her network for advice. She learned that there were many ways to balance work and parenthood, but it required flexibility, communication, and sometimes, tough choices. Some of her colleagues had scaled back their hours or taken on less demanding roles to be more present at home. Others had found ways to integrate work and family life by working from home part-time or adjusting their schedules to fit their needs.

Through these discussions, Jessica realized that maintaining her career while being a present and involved parent would require careful planning and a willingness to adapt. She understood that there might be times when she had to prioritize her family over work or vice versa, but she was determined to find a balance that allowed her to succeed in both areas.

For anyone navigating the transition from full-time work to parenthood, these questions are crucial. How will you manage the demands of your job while being the parent you want to be? What kind of maternity or paternity leave do you have access to, and how will you make the most of it? And how will your long-term career goals fit into your new life as a parent?

These questions don't have easy answers, but by thinking them through and planning ahead, you can create a path that works for you and your family. Balancing work and parenthood is a challenge, but it's also an opportunity to redefine your career and find new ways to achieve your professional and personal goals.

To help you prepare, here are 10 key questions to consider about balancing work and parenthood. After reflecting on these, try the practical exercise to map out your plan for managing your career and family life in a way that feels right for you.

Key Questions:

1. How will we balance work and parenting responsibilities?
2. What are our plans for maternity and paternity leave?
3. Should one of us consider staying home with the baby full-time?
4. How will having a baby impact our long-term career goals?
5. What is our plan for childcare when we return to work?
6. How flexible are our employers with family-related needs?
7. What is our backup plan if one of us needs to work less or

leave work temporarily?

8. How will we manage work-related stress while caring for a newborn?
9. Have we discussed the possibility of changing jobs for better work-life balance?
10. How will we ensure that our careers don't negatively impact our family life?

14

Exercise #5

Practical Exercise:

Create a Work-Family Balance Plan: Sit down with your partner and discuss your work schedules, maternity/paternity leave options, and career goals. Outline a plan for how you will manage your work and parenting responsibilities, including who will handle daily tasks like childcare, drop-offs, and pick-ups. Consider what adjustments might be needed in your work life, such as flexible hours, remote work options, or even a temporary reduction in hours. Write down any potential challenges you anticipate and brainstorm solutions together. This plan will help you both stay on the same page and be better prepared for balancing work and parenthood.

Chapter 6: Living Arrangements

Sophie and Daniel had lived in their cozy apartment for five years. It was the perfect size for the two of them—a charming one-bedroom with a small balcony overlooking the park. They loved their neighborhood, with its tree-lined streets, quaint cafes, and the convenience of being close to work and friends. But when they found out they were expecting a baby, they began to wonder if their beloved apartment would still be suitable for their growing family.

As they sat together in their living room one evening, Sophie looked around and sighed. "Where are we going to put the baby?" she asked, voicing the concern that had been on her mind for weeks. The apartment was already filled with their things, and the idea of squeezing a crib, baby clothes, and all the other necessities into their small space felt overwhelming.

Daniel nodded in agreement. He had been thinking the same thing. "Do you think we need to move?" he asked, though the thought of leaving their neighborhood made him uneasy. They both loved their home, but they also knew that having a baby would change their needs in ways they hadn't fully considered.

The next weekend, they decided to take a closer look at their living situation. They measured the bedroom to see if they could fit a crib next to their bed, and they realized it would be a tight squeeze. They also noticed that their apartment, which had always seemed spacious enough, suddenly felt cramped when they imagined adding baby gear into the mix.

Sophie and Daniel began to explore their options. Should they move to a bigger place? Could they afford a larger apartment or even a house? Or could they make their current space work with some creative rearranging? These questions weighed heavily on their minds as they considered what was best for their future family.

They started by making a list of what they needed in a home now that they were expecting a baby. More space was at the top of the list, but they also wanted to stay in a safe, family-friendly neighborhood with good schools nearby. They considered the importance of having outdoor space, like a backyard or a park within walking distance, where their child could play. Proximity to work and family also played a significant role in their decision-making process.

As they explored potential new homes, Sophie and Daniel quickly realized that finding the perfect place within their budget wouldn't be easy. They visited several apartments and houses, but nothing seemed to tick all the boxes. Some places were spacious but far from their favorite neighborhood. Others were close by but too expensive or in need of significant renovations. The more they looked, the more they realized that they might have to compromise on some of their desires.

At the same time, they revisited the idea of staying in their current apartment. They considered how they could make the space more baby-friendly—perhaps by decluttering, investing in multifunctional furniture, or converting the living room into a dual-purpose nursery. It wouldn't be ideal, but it could be a workable solution, at least for the first year or two.

Throughout this process, Sophie and Daniel learned that choosing the right living arrangements wasn't just about finding the biggest or newest place. It was about creating a home that felt safe, comfortable, and suitable for their new life as parents. They realized that whether they stayed in their cozy apartment or moved to a bigger place, the most important thing was that they felt at ease and prepared for the changes that lay ahead.

If you're preparing to welcome a baby into your home, you may find yourself asking similar questions. Is your current home baby-friendly? Do you have enough space for all the baby essentials? And if not, what are your options? Moving to a new home is a big decision, but so is making your current space work for your growing family.

These are important questions to consider as you plan for your new life as a parent. Your living arrangements will play a significant role in your day-to-day life with a baby, so it's crucial to think through your options and make choices that will support your family's well-being.

To help you get started, here are 10 key questions to consider about your living arrangements. After reflecting on these, try the practical exercise to assess your current home and explore your options for creating a baby-friendly environment.

Key Questions:

1. Is our current home suitable for raising a child?
2. Do we need to move to a larger home or a different neighborhood?
3. How baby-proof is our home, and what changes do we need to make?
4. Do we have a safe and comfortable space for the baby to sleep?
5. Is our home close to good schools and childcare facilities?
6. How will we arrange the baby's nursery or sleeping area?
7. What are the pros and cons of living near family?
8. Should we consider relocating closer to work to reduce commute time?
9. How will our current living situation impact our child's social life and friendships?
10. Do we have access to parks, playgrounds, and outdoor spaces for the baby?

16

Exercise #6

Practical Exercise:

Assess Your Home's Baby-Friendliness: Take a walk through your home with fresh eyes, imagining what it will be like with a baby. Start by evaluating the space where the baby will sleep—will it be in your bedroom or a separate nursery? Measure the space and think about where you will place the crib, changing table, and other essentials. Next, consider safety—are there any hazards like sharp corners, uncovered outlets, or unstable furniture? Finally, think about storage—where will you keep diapers, clothes, toys, and other baby items? Make a list of any changes or upgrades you'll need to make, and start planning how you will prepare your home for your new arrival. If you're considering moving, use this exercise to identify what features are most important in a new home.

17

Chapter 7: Emotional Preparedness

Isabella had always been a confident, organized person. She prided herself on her ability to juggle a busy career, maintain strong friendships, and still find time for self-care. But when she found out she was pregnant, she started to feel an unexpected wave of anxiety. As much as she wanted to be a mother, she couldn't shake the worry that she wasn't emotionally ready for the challenges that lay ahead.

Late one night, Isabella found herself wide awake, her mind racing with thoughts of what life would be like after the baby arrived. She had heard the stories from friends—about the sleepless nights, the endless crying, the overwhelming sense of responsibility. Would she be able to handle it all? What if she didn't bond with her baby right away? And how would she cope with the inevitable stress and exhaustion?

These thoughts filled her with doubt, something she wasn't used to feeling. Normally, Isabella would approach a challenge with a plan and a checklist, but this time, the uncertainty felt too big to manage. She decided it was time to talk to someone who could help her navigate these feelings.

The next day, Isabella called her sister, Maria, who was already a mother of two. Maria had always been a source of wisdom and comfort, and Isabella hoped she could offer some reassurance. As they chatted over the phone, Maria listened patiently to Isabella's concerns. "It's completely normal to feel this way," Maria said gently. "Becoming a parent is a huge emotional shift. But you don't have to do it alone, and it's okay to ask for help."

Maria's words gave Isabella some comfort, but she knew she needed to take action to feel more emotionally prepared. She started by researching the emotional challenges of parenting. She read about postpartum depression, the baby blues, and the common stresses that new parents face. This information helped her understand that her worries were valid and that many new parents experience similar feelings.

But knowledge alone wasn't enough. Isabella realized she needed to develop strategies to manage her emotions and maintain her mental health. She started by building a support network, reaching out to friends who were parents and asking them about their experiences. She also made an appointment with a therapist to discuss her anxieties and learn coping mechanisms.

One of the biggest insights Isabella gained from these conversations was the importance of self-compassion. She had always set high standards for herself, but she began to understand that parenting would require her to be more forgiving of her own imperfections. She would have to learn to be okay with not having all the answers and to give herself grace during the tough moments.

Isabella also began to explore mindfulness and relaxation techniques. She started practicing meditation, which helped her stay grounded when her thoughts started to spiral. She also made a commitment to keep up with activities that brought her joy, like reading and taking long walks, even after the baby arrived. These small acts of self-care became essential parts of her emotional preparedness plan.

As the months went by, Isabella felt more at ease with the idea of becoming a mother. She knew there would be challenging days—days when she felt overwhelmed or unsure—but she also felt more equipped to handle those moments. She had built a toolbox of emotional resources, and she knew she could rely on her support network when things got tough.

For anyone preparing for parenthood, emotional readiness is just as important as physical and financial preparation. It's essential to ask yourself whether you're ready to face the emotional challenges of parenting, how you'll deal with stress, and what steps you can take to maintain your mental health. These questions are key to ensuring that you can approach parenting with resilience and confidence.

As you consider your emotional preparedness, remember that it's okay to feel uncertain or anxious. The important thing is to take steps to address those feelings and to build a support system that can help you through the journey. Emotional preparedness is not about being perfect; it's about being aware of your feelings, seeking help when you need it, and giving yourself the compassion you deserve.

To help you get started, here are 10 key questions to consider about your emotional readiness for parenting. After reflecting on these, try the practical exercise to deepen your understanding of your emotional needs and how you can support yourself through the transition to parenthood.

Key Questions:

1. How do we feel emotionally about becoming parents?
2. Are we prepared to handle the stress and sleep deprivation that comes with a newborn?
3. How will we cope with the potential challenges of postpartum depression or baby blues?
4. How do we plan to maintain our mental health during the early stages of parenting?
5. Are we ready for the changes a baby will bring to our social lives and personal time?
6. How will we manage the pressure of parenting expectations from others?
7. Do we feel ready to handle the responsibility of raising a child?
8. How will we keep communication open about our emotional needs?
9. What support systems do we have in place if we need help?
10. How will we maintain a positive outlook during difficult times?

18

Exercise #7

Practical Exercise:

Create an Emotional Support Plan: Begin by identifying the emotions you expect to face as a new parent—both the positive and the challenging ones. Next, think about the strategies that help you manage stress and maintain your mental health. These might include practices like meditation, journaling, talking to a therapist, or spending time with loved ones. Write down these strategies and consider how you can incorporate them into your daily routine once the baby arrives. Finally, list the people you can turn to for support, whether it's a partner, family member, or friend. Share your plan with your support network so they know how they can help you during this transition. This exercise will help you feel more prepared to face the emotional challenges of parenting with confidence and support.

19

Chapter 8: Childcare and Education

Lily and Mark had always talked about how they would raise their future children, but now that they were expecting, those discussions took on a new urgency. Both were passionate about education, having grown up in families that valued learning and personal development. However, as they began to navigate the maze of options for childcare and education, they realized that making the right choices wasn't as straightforward as they had imagined.

One Saturday morning, as they sat down to breakfast, Lily brought up the topic of daycare. She had been reading about the importance of early childhood education and wanted to make sure their child had the best possible start. "Do you think we should start looking for a daycare now?" she asked, knowing that some of the best centers had long waiting lists. Mark nodded thoughtfully, but he looked a bit uncertain. "I've heard that finding the right place can be tough. What should we even look for?"

This simple question opened the door to a much deeper conversation about their values and expectations when it came to childcare and education. Lily and Mark began to realize that there were many factors to consider—much more than they had initially thought. Would they prefer a daycare that focused on structured learning or one that emphasized play? How important was it to them that their child be in a diverse environment? And how would they balance the costs of high-quality childcare with their budget?

As they discussed these questions, Lily and Mark also began to think about the long-term. They knew that the choices they made in the early years would set the stage for their child's educational journey. This realization led them to explore different schooling options. They debated the merits of public versus private schools, considered the possibility of homeschooling, and even discussed the idea of enrolling their child in a bilingual program to give them a head start in a second language.

But with all these options came uncertainty. Would their child thrive in a traditional school environment, or would they do better in a more flexible setting? How would they ensure that their child received a well-rounded education, including not just academics but also social skills, creativity, and emotional intelligence? The more they thought about it, the more they realized that education was about much more than just what happened in the classroom.

Lily, who had a background in early childhood education, knew that the first few years of a child's life were crucial for their development. She wanted to make sure they chose a daycare that would nurture their child's curiosity and love of learning. Mark, on the other hand, was concerned about the practical aspects—making sure the daycare was safe, conveniently located, and within their budget. They both agreed that finding a balance between these priorities would be key.

To help them make informed decisions, Lily and Mark began visiting different daycare centers and schools in their area. They paid close attention to the environment, the staff's qualifications, and the types of activities offered. They also talked to other parents to get their insights and recommendations. These visits were eye-opening and helped them clarify what they were looking for.

At the same time, they realized that they would need to remain flexible. As much as they wanted to plan every detail of their child's education, they knew that their child's needs and interests might evolve over time. They promised each other that they would stay open to adjusting their plans as their child grew and developed.

For any parent, deciding on childcare and education is one of the most important—and challenging—tasks. It's not just about finding a place to leave your child while you work; it's about laying the foundation for their future learning and development. What kind of environment do you want your child to grow up in? What values do you want their education to reflect? And how will you ensure that your child's educational experience aligns with your hopes and expectations?

These are big questions, and there are no easy answers. But by taking the time to explore your options, understand your priorities, and stay flexible, you can make choices that will help your child thrive both now and in the future.

To help you start thinking about your childcare and education choices, here are 10 key questions to consider. After reflecting on these, try the practical exercise to assess your options and clarify your priorities for your child's early education.

Key Questions:

1. Will we use daycare, a nanny, or family members for childcare?
2. What qualities are most important to us in choosing a childcare provider?
3. How soon should we start looking for and securing childcare?
4. What are our thoughts on early childhood education programs?
5. How do we feel about public versus private schooling?
6. What role will extracurricular activities play in our child's development?
7. How will we handle sick days when childcare isn't available?
8. How important is bilingual or multicultural education to us?
9. What are our thoughts on homeschooling as an option?
10. How will we stay involved in our child's education and school life?

20

Exercise #8

Practical Exercise:

Evaluate Childcare and Education Options: Start by making a list of your top priorities for your child's childcare and education. Consider factors such as location, cost, curriculum, teacher qualifications, and the overall environment. Next, research the options available in your area, including daycare centers, preschools, and other early education programs. If possible, visit these places in person to get a feel for the environment and ask questions. Finally, compare your findings with your priorities and discuss with your partner what would be the best fit for your child. This exercise will help you make an informed decision that aligns with your values and expectations for your child's early years.

21

Chapter 9: Lifestyle Changes

Alex and Taylor had always enjoyed an active lifestyle. Weekends were filled with long hikes, spontaneous road trips, and dinners out with friends. They valued their independence and the freedom to do what they wanted, when they wanted. But as they prepared for the arrival of their first baby, they began to realize that their lives were about to change in ways they hadn't fully considered.

One evening, as they were winding down after a particularly busy day, Taylor turned to Alex and said, "Do you think we'll ever have time for ourselves once the baby comes?" It was a question that had been on both of their minds, but neither had wanted to voice it until now. They both knew that becoming parents would require sacrifices, but they hadn't really thought about how those sacrifices would affect their daily lives.

As they talked, they began to imagine what their new routine might look like. Mornings would likely start much earlier, filled with feeding and diaper changes. The leisurely breakfasts they enjoyed on weekends would be replaced by quick, chaotic meals. And those long hikes they loved? They might have to wait a while before they could strap on a baby carrier and hit the trails again.

Their social life was another big question mark. Alex and Taylor had a close-knit group of friends who they saw regularly, often meeting up for dinners or movie nights. But with a baby, things would undoubtedly change. Would they still be able to meet up with friends as often? Would their friends, many of whom didn't have kids, understand the new demands on their time? And how would they maintain their friendships while adjusting to their new roles as parents?

As they considered these questions, Alex and Taylor realized that they would need to make some changes, not just to their routine, but to their mindset as well. They would have to learn to be more flexible, more willing to let go of their previous expectations, and more open to new ways of enjoying their time together.

One of their biggest concerns was how they would find time for themselves as individuals. Taylor loved painting and often spent hours in the studio, while Alex was an avid cyclist, enjoying long solo rides on weekends. Both of them found these activities essential for their well-being, but they worried that they wouldn't have the time or energy to keep them up once the baby arrived.

To address this, they decided to make a plan. They agreed to take turns giving each other time off—an hour here, a morning there—so that they could continue to pursue their hobbies. They also talked about the importance of staying connected as a couple, even if it meant scheduling date nights at home after the baby was asleep.

As they continued to discuss their upcoming lifestyle changes, Alex and Taylor started to feel more at ease. They knew that their lives would look different, but they also realized that this new chapter could bring its own joys and opportunities for growth. They would still find time for the things they loved, but they would do so with a new sense of purpose and a deeper connection to each other.

For anyone expecting a baby, it's important to consider how your daily routine, hobbies, and social life will change. How will you adjust to the new demands on your time? What activities are essential for your well-being, and how can you make sure you still have time for them? And how will you maintain your social connections while navigating the challenges of parenthood?

These are important questions to ask yourself as you prepare for the lifestyle changes that come with having a baby. By thinking through these changes ahead of time, you can create a plan that helps you stay balanced, fulfilled, and connected, even as you embrace your new role as a parent.

To help you start thinking about these changes, here are 10 key questions to consider. After reflecting on these, try the practical exercise to map out how you can adjust your routine, maintain your hobbies, and stay connected with friends and family after your baby arrives.

Key Questions:

1. How will our daily routine change with a baby?
2. How will we manage time for our hobbies and interests after the baby arrives?
3. What changes will we need to make to our social lives?
4. How will we maintain friendships and social connections with a baby?

5. How do we plan to make time for exercise and staying active?
6. How will our travel plans and vacation habits change?
7. What adjustments will we need to make to our diet and meal planning?
8. How will we ensure that we get enough rest and relaxation?
9. How will having a baby impact our participation in community or religious activities?
10. How do we feel about the potential changes to our personal freedom and spontaneity?

22

Exercise #9

Practical Exercise:

Plan Your New Routine: Take some time to map out what a typical day might look like once the baby arrives. Consider your morning routine, work schedule, meals, and bedtime. Identify where your biggest challenges might be—whether it's finding time for exercise, staying connected with friends, or simply getting enough sleep. Then, brainstorm solutions together. For example, you might decide to take turns watching the baby so each of you can have some personal time, or you might plan to meet up with friends at more family-friendly hours. Writing down this new routine can help you feel more prepared and give you a clearer picture of how your life will change—and how you can still make time for the things that matter most to you.

23

Chapter 10: Emergency and Contingency Planning

David and Mia were the kind of couple who liked to be prepared for anything. They had always prided themselves on their ability to handle whatever life threw their way, whether it was a flat tire on a road trip or a sudden job change. But now that they were expecting their first child, they realized that there was a whole new level of planning they needed to consider. With a baby on the way, they had to think about emergencies and unexpected situations in a way they never had before.

One evening, as they sat down to dinner, Mia brought up the topic. "What do we do if something goes wrong?" she asked, her voice tinged with concern. David looked up from his plate, sensing the seriousness of her question. "Like what?" he replied, though he already had an idea of where the conversation was headed. "You know," Mia continued, "What if the baby gets sick in the middle of the night? Or what if there's an emergency and we need to leave town quickly? We need a plan."

David nodded, realizing that Mia was right. They had always been good at managing day-to-day challenges, but a baby would bring new kinds of emergencies—ones that required careful thought and preparation. They couldn't afford to be caught off guard when it came to their child's safety and well-being.

The first thing they decided to do was create a list of potential emergencies they might face as new parents. They thought about medical emergencies, like a high fever or an allergic reaction, and how they would respond. They also considered situations like a sudden loss of income or the need to evacuate due to a natural disaster. Each scenario made them realize just how important it was to be prepared.

Next, they discussed the importance of having a strong support system in place. They knew they couldn't do it all on their own, especially in a crisis. David suggested making a list of people they could rely on in an emergency—family members, close friends, and trusted neighbors. Mia agreed and added that they should talk to these people ahead of time, letting them know what kind of help they might need and making sure they were willing to step in if necessary.

As they talked, David and Mia also realized the importance of having an emergency fund. They had always been good about saving money, but now they needed to think about how those savings would be used if something unexpected happened. They decided to set aside a portion of their savings specifically for emergencies related to the baby—medical expenses, unexpected travel, or even just extra help if one of them had to take time off work.

Another key part of their planning involved creating an emergency contact list. They wrote down the phone numbers of their pediatrician, local hospital, and nearby urgent care centers, as well as emergency contacts for both of their workplaces. They also made sure they had a list of any medications or allergies the baby might have, along with their insurance information, all in one easily accessible place.

As they continued to plan, David and Mia felt a sense of relief. They knew they couldn't predict every possible scenario, but by thinking ahead and preparing as much as possible, they felt more confident that they could handle whatever came their way. They understood that emergencies would still be stressful, but having a plan in place would help them stay calm and focused.

For any expectant parents, thinking about emergencies and contingency planning can be daunting, but it's a crucial part of preparing for parenthood. What will you do if your baby has a medical emergency? How will you manage if there's a sudden change in your financial situation? And who can you turn to for help if you need it?

These are important questions to consider as you plan for your new life with a baby. By taking the time to prepare for the unexpected, you can ensure that you're ready to respond quickly and effectively, no matter what challenges arise.

To help you get started, here are 10 key questions to consider about emergency and contingency planning. After reflecting on these, try the practical exercise to create an emergency plan that covers a range of potential scenarios and ensures that you have the support and resources you need.

Key Questions:

1. Do we have a plan in case of a medical emergency during pregnancy or after the baby is born?
2. How will we handle emergency situations with the baby, like illness or accidents?

3. What is our plan if one of us needs to take extended leave from work due to a family emergency?
4. Do we have a trusted person to step in if we need help with the baby unexpectedly?
5. How will we prepare for unexpected financial difficulties, such as job loss or unexpected medical bills?
6. Have we considered who will care for the baby if something happens to both of us?
7. What are our plans for handling a difficult birth or medical complications during delivery?
8. How will we ensure our home is safe and secure for the baby in case of an emergency?
9. Do we have a go-to list of emergency contacts and resources readily available?
10. Have we discussed a will or guardianship plan for our child in case of unforeseen circumstances?

24

Exercise #10

Practical Exercise:

Create an Emergency Plan: Begin by identifying the types of emergencies that could potentially arise before and after the baby is born. For each scenario, outline a clear plan of action, including who to contact, what steps to take, and where to go if necessary. Make sure to include contact information for your pediatrician, local hospital, and any other relevant medical professionals. Also, consider setting up an emergency fund specifically for unexpected expenses related to the baby. Once you've created your plan, review it with your partner and any other key people in your support system to ensure everyone is on the same page. Keep a copy of this plan in an easily accessible place so that you can act quickly if an emergency occurs. This exercise will help you feel more prepared and confident in your ability to handle unexpected situations as a new parent.

25

Now WHAT? You May Ask

So, you've read through the chapters, asked yourself the tough questions, and made plans for everything from finances to childcare to emergency situations. You've taken the time to think deeply about your readiness for this incredible journey of becoming a parent. But now, with all these plans in place, you might be asking yourself, "Now what?"

It's a fair question. After all the preparation, where do you go from here? How do you move from planning to action, from thinking about being a parent to actually becoming one? The answer isn't always simple, but it's worth exploring.

First, let's take a moment to acknowledge what you've accomplished so far. You've done the hard work of preparing yourself mentally, emotionally, and practically for the arrival of your baby. That's no small feat. But now, it's time to shift your focus from preparation to anticipation. You're not just getting ready for a baby—you're about to welcome a new person into your life. That's exciting, isn't it?

As you move forward, consider how you can take everything you've learned and put it into practice. How will you integrate your plans into your daily life? Perhaps it's time to start setting up the nursery, organizing baby supplies, or finalizing your work arrangements. But beyond the practical tasks, think about how you'll begin to embody the mindset of a parent. What kind of parent do you want to be, not just in theory, but in everyday moments?

It's easy to get caught up in the details, but don't forget to focus on the bigger picture. Parenthood isn't just about ticking off a checklist—it's about love, connection, and growth. How will you nurture those aspects in your new family? What small steps can you take now to build a strong foundation of love and support?

And let's be honest—there will be moments when things don't go according to plan. Maybe the baby will arrive earlier than expected, or maybe the parenting style you thought would work perfectly needs some adjustment. That's okay. Flexibility is key. How will you adapt when the unexpected happens? How can you stay grounded and calm, even when things get challenging?

Remember, you're not in this alone. Lean on your support system, whether that's your partner, family, friends, or even a community of fellow parents. How will you reach out for help when you need it? How can you ensure that you're not just prepared to give support, but also to receive it?

As the day of your baby's arrival approaches, you might feel a mix of emotions—excitement, nervousness, maybe even a little fear. That's perfectly normal. It's all part of the journey. How will you embrace these feelings without letting them overwhelm you? How can you focus on the joy and wonder of bringing a new life into the world, while also staying grounded in the reality of what's to come?

In the end, the question of "Now what?" is really about

stepping into the unknown with confidence and openness. You've done everything you can to prepare, and now it's time to trust yourself and your ability to navigate this new chapter. How will you approach this journey with a sense of adventure, knowing that you're ready to face whatever comes your way?

Take a deep breath, and remind yourself that you've got this. You're ready. The path ahead may be full of surprises, but it's also full of incredible moments waiting to be experienced. So, now what? Now, you welcome the journey of parenthood with open arms and an open heart.

Because, at the end of the day, this is just the beginning. And what a beautiful beginning it is.

26

Conclusion

As you reach the end of this book, I want to take a moment to thank you. Thank you for buying this book, for investing your time and energy into reading it, and for taking the steps to prepare yourself for the incredible journey of parenthood. Your willingness to ask the tough questions, reflect deeply, and plan thoughtfully speaks to the kind of parent you already are—a parent who is committed to giving your child the best possible start in life.

Throughout these pages, we've explored everything from financial planning to emotional preparedness, from creating a nurturing home environment to finding balance in your work and personal life. I hope that this book has provided you with the insights and tools you need to feel confident and ready as you step into this new chapter.

But before we part ways, I have one more request. If you found value in this book, if it helped you in any way, I encourage you to leave a review. Your thoughts and feedback are incredibly important, not just to me as the author, but to other readers who may be searching for the same guidance and reassurance that you were.

A review from you can make a real difference. It can help this book reach more people, offering them the support they need as they prepare for parenthood. Your review can be the bridge that connects this important message with those who are looking for it—people who may be feeling uncertain, overwhelmed, or simply eager to learn more.

By sharing your thoughts, you're not just reflecting on your own journey; you're helping to create a community of informed, empowered parents who are ready to face the challenges and joys of raising a child. Your words can inspire others, offering them the encouragement and confidence they need as they navigate this exciting time in their lives.

So, if this book has resonated with you, please take a moment to leave a review. It's a small action, but one that has the power to ripple out and touch the lives of many others.

Thank you again for choosing this book, for trusting me to be part of your journey, and for the care and consideration you've shown in preparing for parenthood. I wish you all the best as you step into this beautiful new chapter of your life. May it be filled with love, laughter, and the joy of watching your family grow.

Remember, you've got this. And you're never alone on this journey.

Warmest regards,

Yakalou

www.ingramcontent.com/pod-product-compliance
Lightning Source LLC
Chambersburg PA
CBHW061305250726

48653CB00002B/795